Meal Frequency

---

3 Meals vs. 6 Meals Per Day

By PROSENCE

Copyright 2018 by Prosence - All rights reserved.

This document is geared towards providing exact and reliable information in regards to the topic and issue covered. The publication is sold with the idea that the publisher is not required to render accounting, officially permitted, or otherwise, qualified services. If advice is necessary, legal or professional, a practiced individual in the profession should be ordered.

- From a Declaration of Principles which was accepted and approved equally by a Committee of the American Bar Association and a Committee of Publishers and Associations.

In no way is it legal to reproduce, duplicate, or transmit any part of this document in either electronic means or in printed format. Recording of this publication is strictly prohibited and any storage of this document is not allowed unless with written permission from the publisher. All rights reserved.

The information provided herein is stated to be truthful and consistent, in that any liability, in terms of inattention or otherwise, by any usage or abuse of any policies, processes, or directions contained within is the solitary and utter responsibility of the recipient reader. Under no circumstances will any legal responsibility or blame be held against the publisher for any reparation, damages, or monetary loss due to the information herein, either directly or indirectly.

Respective authors own all copyrights not held by the publisher.

The information herein is offered for informational purposes solely, and is universal as so. The presentation of the information is without contract or any type of guarantee assurance.

The trademarks that are used are without any consent, and the publication of the trademark is without permission or backing by the trademark owner. All trademarks and brands within this book are for clarifying purposes only and are the owned by the owners themselves, not affiliated with this document.

ABOUT PROSENCE

Our Mission

We are dedicated to guiding, motivating and providing the tools necessary to transform people into the best version of themselves. Our goal is to empower men and women across the globe to realize that physical and mental fitness are not a short-term solution, but a lifetime choice, and to actualize what they have come to understand into a daily routine. We invite you to discover this process for yourself as you join us in the exploration of science-based knowledge that can lead to better health, greater fulfillment and astonishing vitality.

Who is Prosence?

Hi, I'm Antonio Mazzotta - certified Fitness Trainer and health enthusiast, and the founder of Prosence. While I don't think I'll ever turn down mom's homemade pasta and pizza, as an Italian living in Switzerland I've built a life dedicated to health and fitness. Now, I want to share the secrets to my success with you.

I got involved in this industry over 7 years ago, and quickly developed a passion for all things health and fitness. I knew right away that this is what I was born to do and haven't looked back. My days are spent developing new routines, training hard and meeting other fitness-minded and health-conscious individuals. I love working with my clients and coaching about weight training, dieting and healthy lifestyle choices. My number one priority is motivating people to achieve any fitness goal they seek. Whether you're looking to lose fat, get stronger, build muscle or just maintain overall health and vitality - Let's reach your goals together!

My team and I work hard to dispel the health and fitness myths and misinformation clogging the Internet today. We're driven by the desire to offer you a safe and manageable yet powerfully effective path to the best health of your life. Prosence is firmly committed to motivating, inspiring, and educating through the sharing of objective, fact-based health and fitness information that is rooted in science. We give you the tools you need to get in great shape and build a lifetime of good health.

Join us - let's work together to maximize your potential and achieve your optimal self while embracing life to the fullest!

Learn more on our website: www.prosencefitness.com, blog and keep up with the daily education and motivation by liking us on Twitter, Facebook & Instagram @prosencefitness.

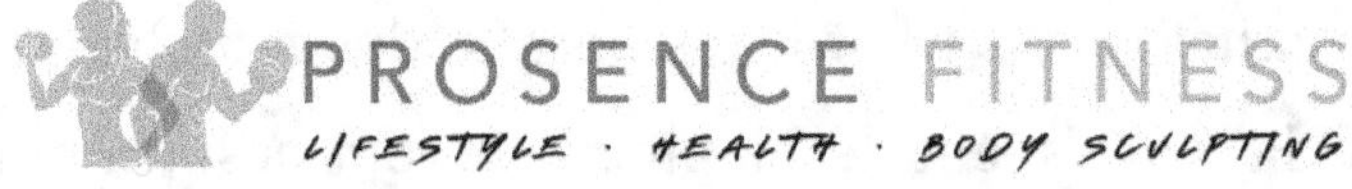

Table of Contents

Introduction

You eat food every day. Or at the very least, almost every day. Otherwise, you wouldn't survive. Food is such a significant part of most people's lives because they spend so much of it either procuring, preparing, or consuming it. If you make a mistake with your diet and the way you eat food that'll have a huge impact on you since you, like almost every other human, have to eat food consistently to survive. It's even more impactful to exercisers and dieters who are attempting to eat food in a specific way to yield a very specific desired outcome. This is why it's important to really make sure you're eating food the best way for you, and at the right frequency.

We here at Prosence are here to help guide you in the exploration of different meal timing strategies, their pros, and their cons. This exploration will mostly relate to health behavior change/psychology and physiological ramifications for the exerciser/lifter.

Is your brain ready to start *processing* a *whole* e-book on this stuff? If so, let's get started.

Chapter 1

Most Common Beliefs About Meal Frequency

There are 4 very commonly used systems that dictate meal frequency. Some people heavily support the consumption of 6 meals scattered evenly throughout the day. Others believe in a traditional approach to eating that involves 3 hardy meals organized in a traditional way (e.g. breakfast upon waking, lunch around noon, and dinner in the evening). Then there is the more unorthodox approach to meal timing called intermittent fasting (sometimes written as "IF"). Finally, some people support the notion that meal frequency and timing are not pertinent to exercise or health. These people typically follow an approach called IIFYM (which is short for "If It Fits In Your Macros"). Though there are 4 common approaches, and they will all be addressed in this section, the 2 most common (6 meals per day and 3 meals per day) will be the focus of the rest of this e-book. IF and IIFYM are important to address briefly given their cultural relevance and extreme takes on meal timing.

Interestingly, all 4 of these major approaches to dieting can lead to positive exercise related adaptations. However, none of them do so optimally. There are very many variables to consider when constructing a perfect diet and most popular diets tend to be a bit negligent in that regard. Each approach has a single minded focus and often hammers that into the head of its followers, rather than promoting a holistic and effective approach that is supported by large bodies of research and professional organizations like the NSCA and ACSM among others. It's easy to market simple solutions to people, which is why the most popular and culturally relevant approaches to meal timing seem to pop up everywhere. But the more nuanced and individualized approaches are the ones that have the greatest efficacy.

Proper meal timing has little to nothing to do with frequency, but really has more to do with the consumption of specific food content (micronutrients and macronutrients) relative to other events in the day and the specific needs and goals of the individuals. However, doing so is a bit complicated to orchestrate without the assistance of a highly trained professional. Because of this, recommendations are often made in regards to meal frequency along with several other supporting suggestions. Some levels of frequency definitely trend towards being superior to others, though whether or not they lead to an optimal diet is based on a bunch of other factors.

Of course different frequencies and styles are best for different people from a psychological and adherence perspective. Regardless of which method trends towards leading to superior physiological adaptations, they all work provided other elements of the diet are in check. Because of this, the most important factor in selecting a diet is whether or not the person that'll be following it can stick with it. If a diet is theoretically superior but someone has too much trouble sticking to it, treating it like it's their only option will hurt them long term. It's best to keep an open mind about meal frequency and go with the best of the options that someone can actually follow.

Perhaps the most common of all approaches in the exercise and diet community involves the consumption of 6 meals per day. These meals are typically evenly spaced and equally calorically dense. If someone plans to consume 2,400 calories in a single day, each meal will have about 400 calories. The meals generally tend to have a balanced composition meaning there are proportionate amount of fat, carbohydrates, and protein in each meal. They also tend to focus on more micronutritionally dense foods. Foods that are dense with micronutrients tend to have high concentrations of vitamins and minerals for the amount of calories they provide.

In general, those that strictly eat 6 meals per day tend to share several common beliefs. Firstly, the followers of this approach often believed that eating consistently throughout the day will lead to an increase in their metabolism and the total amount of calories they burn throughout the day. Eating frequently is seen as a way to stoke the fire, so to speak. It actually requires energy to consume food, and this is often represented by something labeled "the thermic effect of food". Whenever food is consumed, the amount of energy the body expends metabolically increases to handle its absorption and accompanying processes. The more often someone eats, the more of the day will be spent in a state where the body is breaking down food and ergo burning energy.

Secondly, whenever a sizeable amount of carbohydrates is consumed, the body responds by releasing a proportionate amount of insulin. This insulin is intended to clear up the bloodstream of glucose (which increase as a result of eating and especially as a result of carbohydrate consumption), and deliver that glucose to other appropriate tissues in the body. However, insulin also has a secondary effect of being anabolic and anti-catabolic. By having more insulin in the bloodstream, it is harder for the body to break down muscle tissue and easier for it to build it instead. This is very useful for exercisers of all types whether they are attempting to lose fat mass (where maintaining muscle mass is a huge help) or building muscle mass (where it's important to build as much as possible). The thinking of those that consume 6 meals per day generally goes that the more of the day that can be spent with large amounts of insulin released, the more efficient their progress will be.

Thirdly, the anti-catabolic and pro anabolic state is believed by followers of this dietary strategy to be facilitated by simply consuming calories throughout the day irregardless of the source. When a cell is in a state where it is burning more calories than it is consuming, it is considered catabolic and breaks down other tissues in the body to provide the energy it needs to do what it has to. When it's burning less calories than it's consuming, it ends up storing the left over calories to be used for energy to facilitate later processes. Because of this, the thinking of this group is that keeping cells in a fed state where they are not catabolic and breaking down muscle tissue. Or at the very least, making this period last for the greatest percentage of time in the day possible. This is thought to lead to less breakdown of muscle tissue and greater promotion of muscle tissue, even when in a general calorie deficit and losing weight overall.

Taking a completely different approach, those that consume 3 meals per day tend to have a more traditional view of eating.

They believe that eating large amounts of food (typically of different quantities at each meal) will provide the body with all that it needs evenly spaced throughout the day. This group often believes that by consuming larger meals they are better able to stimulate a muscle protein synthesis response by consuming larger meals with larger amounts of protein per meal. They also believe that the believed effects of eating meals gradually throughout the day are a bit overblown and that the same outcomes can be attained by eating regular meals. As an example, the same amount of calories that are consumed will be consumed independent of meal frequency. The thermic effect of food will be essentially the same at the end of the day (because the same food elements require the same amount of energy to break down regardless of when they're consumed and how often) leading to the same net surplus or deficit of calories consumed.

Those that are in the 3 meal per day camp also tend to be more focused on socially normative methods of eating. Because many workplaces and lives are structured around eating only 3 times per day, it is seen as far more convenient and natural to implement when organizing a day. This can make it feel easier for some people to stick with their diet because society naturally supports a 3 meal per day lifestyle.

Intermittent Fasting is a common approach to dieting and involves eating as many meals as one would like within a very short window of time and not eating anything for the rest of the day. There are many different ways to organize an IF diet, but it is very common to see 16 hours of fasting followed by an 8 hour window of eating. This approach attempts to facilitate fat loss by putting the body in a caloric deficit for as long a period as possible before sacrificing too much muscle mass. This group tends to believe that muscle can be built over a long period of time with minimal to not additional fat mass gain because of the dedicated period of the day for fat catabolism. Their views are a bit on the extreme side and often lead to adherence difficulties while also compromising cognitive function during the fasted period of the day. It also tends to lead to unnecessary decreases in training performance and/or amounts of muscle mass loss contrary to the beliefs of its followers. However, if someone can stick to it and it works for them there's no reason to stop.

The final common method of feeding frequency is typically found in IIFYM and claims that timing doesn't matter at all. Meals and food can be consumed at any time of the day yielding a similar effect. This group claims the perfect diet can be achieved by focusing on other variables than timing instead. This claim is definitely inaccurate, but not entirely wrong. Though timing is important, consuming the appropriate type and quantity of macronutrients will have a much larger and more meaningful impact on someone's diet. But, the time food is consumed relative to other events will change the type of adaptations that will occur and their magnitude. So, timing does matter, to some degree.

Chapter 2

Body Composition

As far as body composition goes, changes in this area are primarily a function of the food consumed in the diet rather than the frequency by which it's consumed. Though meal timing alters and affects the mechanisms that impact body composition, it's probably the least important provided at least 3 regularly spaced meals are eaten during the duration of the day. However, assuming all other dietary elements are absolutely perfect and an exerciser is looking to make the most of every slight advantage possible, 6 and 3 meals per day can lead to slightly disparate results.

The most important and impactful period of time for effecting changes in body composition ranges from about an hour or so before beginning a workout until about a few hours after completing a workout. The type of food and amount of food consumed in this period and its timing can have a huge impact on body composition as well as exercise related adaptations, provided food is consumed at all within this timeframe.

Generally speaking, consuming an adequate meal prior to an exercise bout can improve performance during the session and subsequent induce greater levels of positive adaptation post exercise while minimizing negative adaptations like muscle mass loss. Pre workout nutrition should be primarily comprised of carbohydrates, protein, and water. Though a smaller amount of healthy (monounsaturated and/or polyunsaturated) fat should accompany it. This should however be adjusted slightly depending on the training method so that more protein is consumed prior to resistance training and more carbohydrates get consumed prior to cardio. Not eating food beforehand has been demonstrated to significantly reduce performance and potential adaptations post training.

Additionally, consuming a meal immediately after training can facilitate positive adaptations that lead to improvements in body composition by assisting in the maintenance and development of muscle mass. After exercise ends, a protein and carb heavy meal should be consumed to allow for muscles to adapt. Training often leads to a large hormonal response within the body. These hormones circulate and are at their peak concentrations shortly after the conclusion of training, which is why it's important to eat a meal within the "immediately after training" period. By providing anabolic hormones with the dietary substrates they need to build new tissue, more overall muscle mass will be built by the end of the day. Furthermore, exercise often leads to heightened levels of a hormone called cortisol. This is a catabolic hormone and its concentration is highest immediately following the completion of a workout. By eating right after working out, not only is anabolism stimulated, but the catabolic hormone cortisol and its effects are mitigated.

However, aside from the workout period, some studies have demonstrated the need to eat food upon waking and at night before going to sleep because the period of sleep is characterized by high levels of anabolic hormones and tissue repair within the body. This can facilitate recovery from training while also helping to build more overall muscle tissue.

As long as 4 meals are consumed at the specified times of the day mentioned in this section, the timing and frequency of meals won't be all that impactful. Noticeably, this is a problem for the 3 meal per day approach. It simply doesn't allow the flexibility to eat at all times of the day that promote optimal body composition. Of course, the 6 meal per day approach does have this flexibility and room to spare. This makes it the optimal approach for changing and maximizing improvements in body composition. However, the 6 meal per day approach to meal frequency still has to be handled properly. Many people don't consume their 6 meals at adequate times given they equally space out each meal. This is not an optimal approach and instead it is best to consume at least 4 meals at the specified times of morning, pre workout, post workout, and night. Then the final two meals can be interspersed to evenly fill in the biggest time gaps between the other 4.

Chapter 3

Metabolism

The metabolism and the way different meal frequencies effect it is often the first thing people consider when deciding which dietary approach to adopt. Though, interestingly, many who do this misinterpret and misunderstood what the metabolism even is. It is essentially the sum of all chemical reactions and processes within the body. Whenever something happens in the body at a chemical level, it's considered to be a part of the metabolism. If the same foods items are consumed throughout the day when the body is in the same state, the same chemical reactions will occur. If the environment food is consumed in is different, different reactions will occur. The type of reactions that occur will lead to different amounts of calories being burned as well as different types and degrees of adaptation at the cellular level.

Because of the varied times and environments that 3 or 6 meal per day plans can be implemented within, it is impossible to predict the exact effects these approaches would have on the overall metabolism of the body and daily caloric energy expenditure. Instead, it is only possible to consider the way that the distance between meal consumption times impacts the metabolism.

Given the average person is awake for approximately 16 hours each day, and each meal is assumed to be consumed equidistant to one another, those eating 6 meals per day will eat an average of 1 meal every 2.5 or so hours. Those eating 3 meals per day would consume an average of 1 meal every 5 or so hours. However, with those differences in time a similar amount of energy should be burned whether someone eats 3 or 6 meals per day. This would change in favor of an individual eating 6 meals per day burning more if the 6 meals were perfectly (and not evenly) timed as described earlier, because doing so would mean there would be more overall adaptation (which requires excess energy).

Chapter 4

Hunger and Satiety

The interesting thing about hunger as a physiological response is that it is highly regulated by an individual's psyche. Hunger has physiological underpinnings in that it is intended to alert an individual that their body is lacking certain nutrients, yes. However, the perception of hunger and its interpretation is entirely psychological. Even some non-hunger related phenomena related to satiety and eating when anxious or bored are manifested by psychological constructs. Because of this, there are certain tricks that can be used to manage the perception of hunger and desire to consume more food. Though a full exploration of these tricks is outside the scope of this section, one such trick happens to be eating frequently throughout the day.

Eating 6 meals per day can do a significant amount to curb hunger and increase satiety. This is in part due to the relationship between perceived hunger and temporal recency. The more recent it feels like someone ate, the less likely they will be to seek out more food. Eating 6 meals per day does just that. At most dieters will have only eaten several hours earlier, rather than 5+. Additionally, eating at a high frequency can also help curb eating out of boredom or anxiety which will increase satiety. Because these behaviors are linked to neurochemical responses in the brain to the consumption of food, going long periods of time without food creates a greater need for these responses. By eating frequently and thus having a more regular drip of neurochemical responses to food within the brain throughout the day, the urge to induce them through random snacking will decrease.

Though it is generally more helpful to consume 6 meals per day rather than 3 in regards to hunger and satiety, it is also important to consider the habituation that occurs with any meal frequency pattern. If eating the same amount of food at consistently the same times each day (regardless of meal frequency), hunger will set in at the time food is regularly eaten. So, in that regard, both meal frequencies are on equal terms. However, 6 meals per day tends to be superior in most regards. But of course if someone has an easier time adhering to 3 meals per day to manage hunger, and it works for them, it's not harmful to continue with that dietary strategy.

Chapter 5

Protein Synthesis

Muscle protein synthesis is hugely important whenever considering any sort of muscle related adaptation. As discussed earlier, meal timing in this regard is paramount when considered relative to the application time of a bout of exercise training. However, muscle protein synthesis is important to consider from another perspective. The rate and degree of muscle protein synthesis can be influenced by the quantity of protein consumed during any meal as well as the meal's general composition. This is a very important consideration in meal timing given that the 6 meal per day approach leads to lower protein dense meals and the 3 meal per day approach leads to meals with higher protein density.

It is possible to consume an amount of protein per meal that is too low to maximize muscle protein synthesis and thereby compromise results. The amount that should be consumed, at a minimum, usually ranges between 20-35 grams depending on the person, but usually skews towards the high 20s, low 30s. Research in this area has produced mixed results causing there to be a range. It is suggested that this means the prerequisite amount varies depending on individual characteristics. Consuming more protein (within reason) during a meal than the amount needed to maximize the muscle protein synthesis response is usually an okay thing provided the total amount of protein consumed throughout the day doesn't exceed an unhealthy or damaging amount and the dieter is a healthy adult with consent from their dietician.

Unfortunately, whether consuming 3 meals or 6 meals per day will heavily affect muscle protein synthesis is based on the individual person. If someone requires a smaller target of 100 grams of protein per day, they may not be getting the most of their muscle protein synthesis response by eating 6 meals per day. However if someone is much bigger and requires 200 grams of protein per day (very uncommon), they would probably be consuming too much protein per meal by eating just 3 meals per day. For most people though, 6 meals should be the right amount and feel a bit more natural than 3 high protein meals.

Chapter 6

Insulin Response

Insulin is an extremely important hormone. As discussed earlier it has an important role in the promotion of muscle anabolism and the downregulation of muscle catabolism. However, it also plays a role in the onset of type II diabetes mellitus. Though all information and education within this e-book is intended solely for healthy adults and is not to be used to treat or manage a chronic disease, it is still important to consider the implications of reducing the body's sensitivity to insulin.

When someone eats consistently throughout the day they're basically going to flood themselves in a constant sea of insulin. An argument can be made for the benefits this would have more immediately for adaptations to exercise, however it's also important to consider the long run. By being frequently exposed to large amounts of insulin, the body's insulin receptors become less sensitive to it. When this happens on a significant level, type II diabetes mellitus develops and the body ends up having a hard time managing its blood sugar. Because of this risk, always eating many high carb meals throughout the day may not be as advantageous as it initially sounds. This risk factor, however, can be offset by the application of regular cardio. Regularly engaging in aerobically taxing exercise such as running or swimming can help manage blood sugar and thereby assist in limiting the magnitude of constant insulin responses, according to some research.

It is really easy when considering training and dietary strategies to ignore their long term risks. Everything in moderation is fine, but eating too frequently (similar to eating too infrequently) can be bad news. For most people eating 6 meals per day with a reasonable amount of calories and regular exercise shouldn't be any cause for concern. However it's important for risk management to not increase that number of meals by too much while also consuming a high carb diet along with little to no cardio. Ultimately though, most healthy adults should be fine.

Chapter 7

Frequently Asked Questions

I have a chronic disease, does this still apply to me?

Maybe, but it's best to consult a registered dietician in person. Having a chronic disease can completely change what your body needs and the effect that eating in certain ways has on it. No advice within this e-book should be used to treat or manage a chronic disease because that would be dangerous. All information in this e-book is intended for healthy adults. If you are interested in finding out whether or not it is okay to eat a certain way and have a chronic disease, don't turn to online help for dietary advice. Find an in person registered dietician and discuss the issue with them. Of course, exercise is a bit different. If a doctor clears you to exercise or recommends it, consulting with one of our educated and certified personal trainers at Prosence is completely fine.

What if I really want to follow a certain diet like IIFYM or IF?

That's completely okay! The most important thing when it comes to exercise and dieting is picking something that you want to do, that makes you happy, that you can stick to/actually do, and that still accomplished your goals. Two approaches to dieting can accomplish the same end result at different rates, but that doesn't mean the slower path is wrong if it makes you happy or it's the only path you won't fall off of. It's easy to become paralyzed and feel trapped in thinking that you have to eat a very specific certain way, but in reality, you have a few options if you don't mind progress being a little slower and all.

Conclusion

I hope that this in depth review of meal timing strategies will in some aid you in your endeavors. As you become more and more adapted/well trained, smaller considerations such as meal timing will have larger and larger ramifications to your training and potential to adapt further. Understanding the fundamentals should allow you to make informed dietary decisions in your own best interest from this point onward.

Seeing as we've reached the end of our journey, you know what you have to do next. It's time to put this knowledge to good use and plan your daily meals appropriately in order to optimize your progress towards your goals. Now that you won't have any doubt about whether or not your meal timing approach is correct, it should be much easier to stick to it! Good luck out there.

Thank you for purchasing this book, I hope you enjoyed it.

Finally, if you enjoyed this book then I'd like to ask you for a favor. Will you be kind enough to leave a review for this book on Amazon? It would be greatly appreciated!

Don't forget to follow us on Twitter, Facebook & Instagram and visit our website www.prosencefitness.com to get empowered, educated and inspired to become the best version of yourself in life! You deserve it.

References

1. Antonio, J., Kalman, D., Stout, J. R., Greenwood, M., Willoughby, D. S., & Haff, G. G. (Eds.). (2009). Essentials of sports nutrition and supplements. Springer Science & Business Media.

2. Bandin, C., Scheer, F. A. J. L., Luque, A. J., Avila-Gandia, V., Zamora, S., Madrid, J. A., ... & Garaulet, M. (2015). Meal timing affects glucose tolerance, substrate oxidation and circadian-related variables: a randomized, crossover trial. International journal of obesity, 39(5), 828.

3. Bellisle, F., McDevitt, R., & Prentice, A. M. (1997). Meal frequency and energy balance. British Journal of Nutrition, 77(S1), S57-S70.

4. FAíBRY, P. A. V. E. L., & Tepperman, J. (1970). Meal frequency—a possible factor in human pathology. The American journal of clinical nutrition, 23(8), 1059-1068.

5. Farshchi, H. R., Taylor, M. A., & Macdonald, I. A. (2004). Regular meal frequency creates more appropriate insulin sensitivity and lipid profiles compared with irregular meal frequency in healthy lean women. European journal of clinical nutrition, 58(7), 1071.

6. Haff, G., & Triplett, N. T. (2016). Essentials of strength training and conditioning. Champaign, IL: Human Kinetics.

7. Hulmi, J. J., Laakso, M., Mero, A. A., Häkkinen, K., Ahtiainen, J. P., & Peltonen, H. (2015). The effects of whey protein with or without carbohydrates on resistance training adaptations. Journal of the International Society of Sports Nutrition, 12(1), 48.

8. Jakubowicz, D., Froy, O., Wainstein, J., & Boaz, M. (2012). Meal timing and composition influence ghrelin levels, appetite scores and weight loss maintenance in overweight and obese adults. Steroids, 77(4), 323-331.

9. Kerksick, C., Harvey, T., Stout, J., Campbell, B., Wilborn, C., Kreider, R., ... & Ivy, J. L. (2008). International Society of Sports Nutrition position stand: nutrient

timing. Journal of the International Society of Sports Nutrition, 5(1), 17.

10. Klempel, M. C., Kroeger, C. M., Bhutani, S., Trepanowski, J. F., & Varady, K. A. (2012). Intermittent fasting combined with calorie restriction is effective for weight loss and cardio-protection in obese women. Nutrition journal, 11(1), 98.

11. Mattson, M. P., Allison, D. B., Fontana, L., Harvie, M., Longo, V. D., Malaisse, W. J., ... & Seyfried, T. N. (2014). Meal frequency and timing in health and disease. Proceedings of the National Academy of Sciences, 111(47), 16647-16653.

12. Maughan, R. J. (1999). Role of micronutrients in sport and physical activity. British Medical Bulletin, 55(3), 683-690.

13. Morgan, L. M., Shi, J. W., Hampton, S. M., & Frost, G. (2012). Effect of meal timing and glycaemic index on glucose control and insulin secretion in healthy volunteers. British Journal of Nutrition, 108(7), 1286-1291.

14. Phillips, S. M. (2011). The science of muscle hypertrophy: making dietary protein count. Proceedings of the Nutrition Society, 70(1), 100-103.

15. Phillips, S. M., & Van Loon, L. J. (2011). Dietary protein for athletes: from requirements to optimum adaptation. Journal of sports sciences, 29(sup1), S29-S38.

16. Reid, K. J., Baron, K. G., & Zee, P. C. (2014). Meal timing influences daily caloric intake in healthy adults. Nutrition Research, 34(11), 930-935.

17. Schoenfeld, B. J., Aragon, A. A., & Krieger, J. W. (2013). The effect of protein timing on muscle strength and hypertrophy: a meta-analysis. Journal of the International Society of Sports Nutrition, 10(1), 53.

18. Smeets, A. J., & Westerterp-Plantenga, M. S. (2008). Acute effects on metabolism and appetite profile of one meal difference in the lower range of meal frequency. British journal of nutrition, 99(6), 1316-1321.

19. Stark, M., Lukaszuk, J., Prawitz, A., & Salacinski, A. (2012). Protein timing and its effects on muscular hypertrophy and strength in individuals engaged in weight-training. Journal of the International Society of Sports Nutrition, 9(1), 54.

20. Thomas, D. T., Erdman, K. A., & Burke, L. M. (2016). American College of Sports Medicine Joint Position Statement. Nutrition and Athletic Performance. Medicine and science in sports and exercise, 48(3), 543-568.